This Journal Belongs To

_____

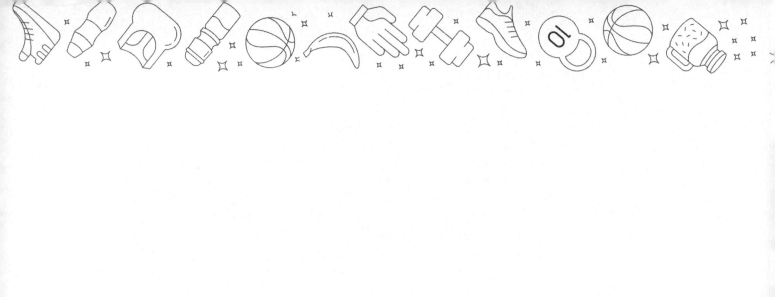

Want free goodies?!

We want to offer you some exclusive freebies and a weight loss hack
that will help you achieve your goals even faster.
Simply visit our website below ⬇️

SCAN THE QR CODE OR VISIT:

www.theplanetnutrition.com

My Starting Measurements

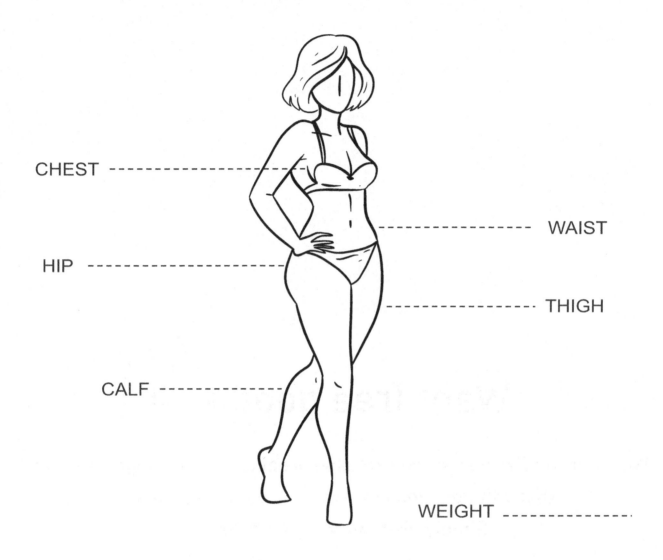

CHEST --------------

HIP --------------

CALF --------------

WAIST --------------

THIGH --------------

WEIGHT --------------

⭐ Things I like about my Body

....

....

⭐ Things I'd like to improve

....

....

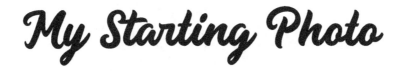

My Starting Photo

Glue in a photo of yourself, not the perfect one!
So you can look back at it at the end of your journey to be amazed!

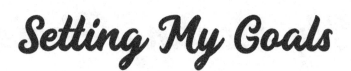

Setting My Goals

Goal 1

....

....

Why do you Want to Achieve This Goal ?

....

....

Goal 2

....

....

Why do you Want to Achieve This Goal ?

....

....

Goal 3

....

....

Why do you Want to Achieve This Goal ?

....

....

Progress Tracker

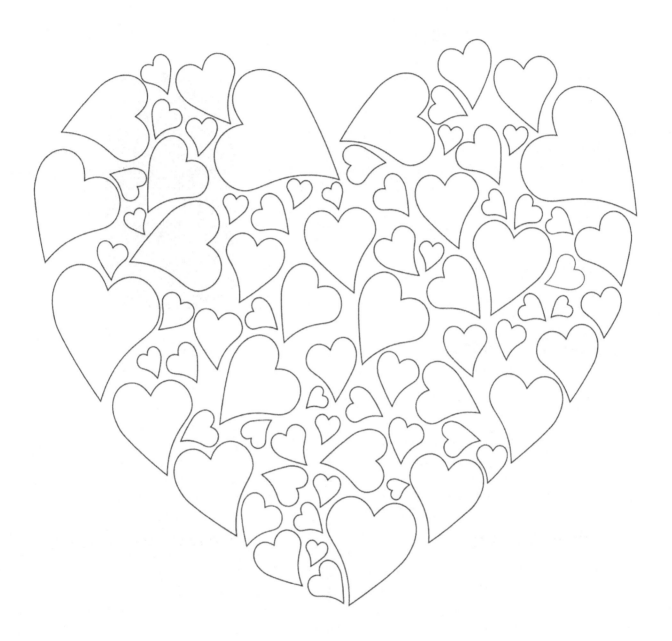

->>>>> COLOR YOUR DAY <<<<<-

RED
If Completed

Yellow
If Completed
partially
(e.g. missed out fitness log,
water intake etc.)

Black
If Skipped

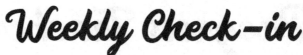

Weekly Check-in

Weekly Goals

☐ _____
_____

☐ _____
_____

☐ _____
_____

Measurements

CHEST	
WAIST	
HIPS	
THIGH	
CALF	
WEIGHT	

Good Habits to Build

_____
_____
_____
_____

Bad Habits to Cut

_____
_____
_____
_____

How I'm Feeling

_____
_____
_____
_____

Reasons to keep Going

_____
_____
_____
_____

CALORIES	MONDAY	TUESDAY	WEDNESDAY	THURSDAY	FRIDAY	SATURDAY	SUNDAY
TOTAL							
GOAL							

Date: ....   Weight: ....

Breakfast

_____
_____
_____
_____

CALORIES ....

Lunch

_____
_____
_____
_____

CALORIES ....

Dinner

_____
_____
_____
_____

CALORIES ....

Snacks

_____
_____
_____
_____

CALORIES ....

Water

Caffeine

Sleep

Steps

ACTIVITY/EXERCISE	AMOUNT	NOTES

My Mood is

_____
_____
_____

Ideas for Tomorrow

_____
_____
_____

First Bite

Last Bite

Daily Calories

Date: ....   **Weight:** ....

Breakfast

_____
_____
_____
_____

CALORIES ....

Lunch

_____
_____
_____
_____

CALORIES ....

Dinner

_____
_____
_____
_____

CALORIES ....

Snacks

_____
_____
_____
_____

CALORIES ....

Water

Caffeine

Sleep

Steps

ACTIVITY/EXERCISE	AMOUNT	NOTES

First Bite

Last Bite

My Mood is

_____
_____
_____

Ideas for Tomorrow

_____
_____
_____

Daily Calories

Date: ....   **Weight:** ....

Breakfast

_____
_____
_____
_____

CALORIES ....

Lunch

_____
_____
_____
_____

CALORIES ....

Dinner

_____
_____
_____
_____

CALORIES ....

Snacks

_____
_____
_____
_____

CALORIES ....

Water

Caffeine

Sleep

Steps

ACTIVITY/EXERCISE	AMOUNT	NOTES

First Bite

Last Bite

My Mood is

_____
_____
_____

Ideas for Tomorrow

_____
_____
_____

Daily Calories

Date: .... Weight: ....

Breakfast

_____
_____
_____
_____

CALORIES ....

Lunch

_____
_____
_____
_____

CALORIES ....

Dinner

_____
_____
_____
_____

CALORIES ....

Snacks

_____
_____
_____
_____

CALORIES ....

Water

Caffeine

Sleep

Steps

ACTIVITY/EXERCISE	AMOUNT	NOTES

My Mood is

_____
_____
_____

Ideas for Tomorrow

_____
_____
_____
_____

First Bite

Last Bite

Daily Calories

Date:................. Weight:.................

Breakfast

_____
_____
_____
_____

CALORIES ....

Dinner

_____
_____
_____
_____

CALORIES ....

Lunch

_____
_____
_____
_____

CALORIES ....

Snacks

_____
_____
_____
_____

CALORIES ....

Water

Caffeine

Sleep

Steps

ACTIVITY/EXERCISE	AMOUNT	NOTES

My Mood is

_____
_____
_____

Ideas for Tomorrow

_____
_____
_____

First Bite

Last Bite

Daily Calories

Date: ....

Weight: ....

Breakfast

_____

_____

_____

_____

CALORIES ....

Lunch

_____

_____

_____

_____

CALORIES ....

Water

Caffeine

Dinner

_____

_____

_____

_____

CALORIES ....

Snacks

_____

_____

_____

_____

CALORIES ....

Sleep

Steps

ACTIVITY/EXERCISE	AMOUNT	NOTES

First Bite

Last Bite

My Mood is

_____

_____

_____

Ideas for Tomorrow

_____

_____

_____

Daily Calories

Date:.................   Weight:.................

Breakfast

_____
_____
_____
_____

CALORIES ....

Lunch

_____
_____
_____
_____

CALORIES ....

Dinner

_____
_____
_____
_____

CALORIES ....

Snacks

_____
_____
_____
_____

CALORIES ....

Water

Caffeine

Sleep

Steps

ACTIVITY/EXERCISE	AMOUNT	NOTES

My Mood is

_____
_____
_____

Ideas for Tomorrow

_____
_____
_____

First Bite

Last Bite

Daily Calories

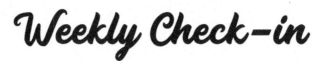

Weekly Check-in

Weekly Goals

☐ _____
_____

☐ _____
_____

☐ _____
_____

Measurements

CHEST	
WAIST	
HIPS	
THIGH	
CALF	
WEIGHT	

Good Habits to Build

_____
_____
_____
_____

Bad Habits to Cut

_____
_____
_____
_____

How I'm Feeling

_____
_____
_____
_____

Reasons to keep Going

_____
_____
_____
_____

CALORIES	MONDAY	TUESDAY	WEDNESDAY	THURSDAY	FRIDAY	SATURDAY	SUNDAY
TOTAL							
GOAL							

Date: .... Weight: ....

Breakfast

_____
_____
_____
_____

CALORIES ....

Lunch

_____
_____
_____
_____

CALORIES ....

Water

Caffeine

Dinner

_____
_____
_____
_____

CALORIES ....

Snacks

_____
_____
_____
_____

CALORIES ....

Sleep

Steps

ACTIVITY/EXERCISE	AMOUNT	NOTES

First Bite

Last Bite

My Mood is

_____
_____
_____

Ideas for Tomorrow

_____
_____
_____

Daily Calories

Date: .... **Weight:** ....

Breakfast

_____
_____
_____
_____

CALORIES ....

Lunch

_____
_____
_____
_____

CALORIES ....

Dinner

_____
_____
_____
_____

CALORIES ....

Snacks

_____
_____
_____
_____

CALORIES ....

Water

Caffeine

Sleep

Steps

ACTIVITY/EXERCISE	AMOUNT	NOTES

First Bite

Last Bite

My Mood is

_____
_____
_____

Ideas for Tomorrow

_____
_____
_____

Daily Calories

Date: ....

Weight: ....

Breakfast

_____
_____
_____
_____

CALORIES ....

Dinner

_____
_____
_____
_____

CALORIES ....

Lunch

_____
_____
_____
_____

CALORIES ....

Snacks

_____
_____
_____
_____

CALORIES ....

Water

Caffeine

Sleep

Steps

ACTIVITY/EXERCISE	AMOUNT	NOTES

My Mood is

_____
_____
_____

Ideas for Tomorrow

_____
_____
_____
_____

First Bite

Last Bite

Daily Calories

Date:................... Weight:..................

Breakfast

_____
_____
_____
_____

CALORIES ....

Lunch

_____
_____
_____
_____

CALORIES ....

Dinner

_____
_____
_____
_____

CALORIES ....

Snacks

_____
_____
_____
_____

CALORIES ....

Water

Caffeine

Sleep

Steps

ACTIVITY/EXERCISE	AMOUNT	NOTES

First Bite

Last Bite

My Mood is

_____
_____
_____

Ideas for Tomorrow

_____
_____
_____

Daily Calories

Date: ....   Weight: ....

Breakfast

_____
_____
_____
_____

CALORIES ....

Dinner

_____
_____
_____
_____

CALORIES ....

Lunch

_____
_____
_____
_____

CALORIES ....

Snacks

_____
_____
_____
_____

CALORIES ....

Water

Caffeine

Sleep

Steps

ACTIVITY/EXERCISE	AMOUNT	NOTES

First Bite

Last Bite

My Mood is

_____
_____
_____

Ideas for Tomorrow

_____
_____
_____

Daily Calories

Date: ....   **Weight:** ....

Breakfast

_____
_____
_____
_____
_____

CALORIES ....

Lunch

_____
_____
_____
_____
_____

CALORIES ....

Water

Caffeine

Dinner

_____
_____
_____
_____

CALORIES ....

Snacks

_____
_____
_____
_____

CALORIES ....

Sleep

Steps

ACTIVITY/EXERCISE	AMOUNT	NOTES

First Bite

Last Bite

My Mood is

_____
_____
_____
_____

Ideas for Tomorrow

_____
_____
_____
_____

Daily Calories

Date: ....   Weight: ....

Breakfast

_____
_____
_____
_____

CALORIES ....

Lunch

_____
_____
_____
_____

CALORIES ....

Dinner

_____
_____
_____
_____

CALORIES ....

Snacks

_____
_____
_____
_____

CALORIES ....

Water

Caffeine

Sleep

Steps

ACTIVITY/EXERCISE	AMOUNT	NOTES

My Mood is

_____
_____
_____

Ideas for Tomorrow

_____
_____
_____

First Bite

Last Bite

Daily Calories

Weekly Check-in

Weekly Goals

☐ _____
  _____

☐ _____
  _____

☐ _____
  _____

Measurements

CHEST	
WAIST	
HIPS	
THIGH	
CALF	
WEIGHT	

Good Habits to Build

_____
_____
_____
_____

Bad Habits to Cut

_____
_____
_____
_____

How I'm Feeling

_____
_____
_____
_____

Reasons to keep Going

_____
_____
_____
_____

CALORIES	MONDAY	TUESDAY	WEDNESDAY	THURSDAY	FRIDAY	SATURDAY	SUNDAY
TOTAL							
GOAL							

Date: ....

Weight: ....

Breakfast

_____
_____
_____
_____

CALORIES ....

Lunch

_____
_____
_____
_____

CALORIES ....

Water

Caffeine

Dinner

_____
_____
_____
_____

CALORIES ....

Snacks

_____
_____
_____
_____

CALORIES ....

Sleep

Steps

ACTIVITY/EXERCISE	AMOUNT	NOTES

First Bite

Last Bite

My Mood is

_____
_____
_____

Ideas for Tomorrow

_____
_____
_____

Daily Calories

Date: .... **Weight:** ....

Breakfast
_____
_____
_____
_____

CALORIES ....

Lunch
_____
_____
_____
_____

CALORIES ....

Dinner
_____
_____
_____
_____

CALORIES ....

Snacks
_____
_____
_____
_____

CALORIES ....

Water

Caffeine

Sleep

Steps

ACTIVITY/EXERCISE	AMOUNT	NOTES

First Bite

Last Bite

My Mood is
_____
_____
_____

Ideas for Tomorrow
_____
_____
_____

Daily Calories

Date: ....   Weight: ....

Breakfast

_____
_____
_____
_____

CALORIES ....

Dinner

_____
_____
_____
_____

CALORIES ....

Lunch

_____
_____
_____
_____

CALORIES ....

Snacks

_____
_____
_____
_____

CALORIES ....

Water

Caffeine

Sleep

Steps

ACTIVITY/EXERCISE	AMOUNT	NOTES

My Mood is

_____
_____
_____

Ideas for Tomorrow

_____
_____
_____

First Bite

Last Bite

Daily Calories

Date:..................   **Weight:**..................

Breakfast

_____
_____
_____
_____
_____

CALORIES ....

Lunch

_____
_____
_____
_____
_____

CALORIES ....

Water

Caffeine

Dinner

_____
_____
_____
_____
_____

CALORIES ....

Snacks

_____
_____
_____
_____
_____

CALORIES ....

Sleep

Steps

ACTIVITY/EXERCISE	AMOUNT	NOTES

First Bite

Last Bite

My Mood is

_____
_____
_____

Ideas for Tomorrow

_____
_____
_____

Daily Calories

Date: .... Weight: ....

Breakfast

_____
_____
_____
_____

CALORIES ....

Lunch

_____
_____
_____
_____

CALORIES ....

Water

(10 glasses)

Caffeine

Dinner

_____
_____
_____
_____

CALORIES ....

Snacks

_____
_____
_____
_____

CALORIES ....

Sleep

Steps

ACTIVITY/EXERCISE	AMOUNT	NOTES

First Bite

Last Bite

My Mood is

_____
_____
_____

Ideas for Tomorrow

_____
_____
_____

Daily Calories

Date: ....

Weight: ....

Breakfast

_____

_____

_____

_____

CALORIES ....

Lunch

_____

_____

_____

_____

CALORIES ....

Dinner

_____

_____

_____

_____

CALORIES ....

Snacks

_____

_____

_____

_____

CALORIES ....

Water

Caffeine

Sleep

Steps

ACTIVITY/EXERCISE	AMOUNT	NOTES

My Mood is

_____

_____

_____

Ideas for Tomorrow

_____

_____

_____

First Bite

Last Bite

Daily Calories

Date: ....   Weight: ....

Breakfast

_____
_____
_____
_____

CALORIES ....

Lunch

_____
_____
_____
_____

CALORIES ....

Water

Caffeine

Dinner

_____
_____
_____
_____

CALORIES ....

Snacks

_____
_____
_____
_____

CALORIES ....

Sleep

Steps

ACTIVITY/EXERCISE	AMOUNT	NOTES

First Bite

Last Bite

My Mood is

_____
_____
_____

Ideas for Tomorrow

_____
_____
_____

Daily Calories

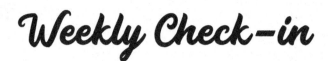

Weekly Check-in

Weekly Goals

☐ _____
_____

☐ _____
_____

☐ _____
_____

Measurements

CHEST	
WAIST	
HIPS	
THIGH	
CALF	
WEIGHT	

Good Habits to Build

_____
_____
_____
_____

Bad Habits to Cut

_____
_____
_____
_____

How I'm Feeling

_____
_____
_____
_____

Reasons to keep Going

_____
_____
_____
_____

CALORIES	MONDAY	TUESDAY	WEDNESDAY	THURSDAY	FRIDAY	SATURDAY	SUNDAY
TOTAL							
GOAL							

Date: ....   Weight: ....

Breakfast

_____
_____
_____
_____
_____

CALORIES ....

Lunch

_____
_____
_____
_____
_____

CALORIES ....

Water

Dinner

_____
_____
_____
_____
_____

CALORIES ....

Snacks

_____
_____
_____
_____
_____

CALORIES ....

Caffeine

Sleep

Steps

ACTIVITY/EXERCISE	AMOUNT	NOTES

First Bite

Last Bite

My Mood is

_____
_____
_____

Ideas for Tomorrow

_____
_____
_____

Daily Calories

Date: .... Weight: ....

Breakfast

_____
_____
_____
_____

CALORIES ....

Dinner

_____
_____
_____
_____

CALORIES ....

Lunch

_____
_____
_____
_____

CALORIES ....

Snacks

_____
_____
_____
_____

CALORIES ....

Water

Caffeine

Sleep

Steps

ACTIVITY/EXERCISE	AMOUNT	NOTES

My Mood is

_____
_____
_____

Ideas for Tomorrow

_____
_____
_____

First Bite

Last Bite

Daily Calories

Date: ....

Weight: ....

Breakfast

_____
_____
_____
_____

CALORIES ....

Lunch

_____
_____
_____
_____

CALORIES ....

Water

Caffeine

Dinner

_____
_____
_____
_____

CALORIES ....

Snacks

_____
_____
_____
_____

CALORIES ....

Sleep

Steps

ACTIVITY/EXERCISE	AMOUNT	NOTES

First Bite

Last Bite

My Mood is

_____
_____
_____

Ideas for Tomorrow

_____
_____
_____

Daily Calories

Date:................. Weight:.................

Breakfast

_____
_____
_____
_____

CALORIES ....

Dinner

_____
_____
_____
_____

CALORIES ....

Lunch

_____
_____
_____
_____

CALORIES ....

Snacks

_____
_____
_____
_____

CALORIES ....

Water

Caffeine

Sleep

Steps

ACTIVITY/EXERCISE	AMOUNT	NOTES

My Mood is

_____
_____
_____

Ideas for Tomorrow

_____
_____
_____

First Bite

Last Bite

Daily Calories

Date: ....   Weight: ....

Breakfast

_____
_____
_____
_____

CALORIES ....

Lunch

_____
_____
_____
_____

CALORIES ....

Water

Caffeine

Dinner

_____
_____
_____
_____

CALORIES ....

Snacks

_____
_____
_____
_____

CALORIES ....

Sleep

Steps

ACTIVITY/EXERCISE	AMOUNT	NOTES

First Bite

My Mood is

_____
_____
_____

Ideas for Tomorrow

_____
_____
_____

Last Bite

Daily Calories

Date: .... Weight: ....

Breakfast

_____
_____
_____
_____

CALORIES ....

Lunch

_____
_____
_____
_____

CALORIES ....

Water

Caffeine

Dinner

_____
_____
_____
_____

CALORIES ....

Snacks

_____
_____
_____
_____

CALORIES ....

Sleep

Steps

ACTIVITY/EXERCISE	AMOUNT	NOTES

First Bite

Last Bite

My Mood is

_____
_____
_____

Ideas for Tomorrow

_____
_____
_____

Daily Calories

Date: ....

Weight: ....

Breakfast

_____
_____
_____
_____

CALORIES ....

Lunch

_____
_____
_____
_____

CALORIES ....

Water

Caffeine

Dinner

_____
_____
_____
_____

CALORIES ....

Snacks

_____
_____
_____
_____

CALORIES ....

Sleep

Steps

ACTIVITY/EXERCISE	AMOUNT	NOTES

My Mood is

_____
_____
_____

Ideas for Tomorrow

_____
_____
_____

First Bite

Last Bite

Daily Calories

Weekly Check-in

Weekly Goals

☐ _____
_____

☐ _____
_____

☐ _____
_____

Measurements

CHEST	
WAIST	
HIPS	
THIGH	
CALF	
WEIGHT	

Good Habits to Build

_____
_____
_____
_____

Bad Habits to Cut

_____
_____
_____
_____

How I'm Feeling

_____
_____
_____
_____

Reasons to keep Going

_____
_____
_____
_____

CALORIES	MONDAY	TUESDAY	WEDNESDAY	THURSDAY	FRIDAY	SATURDAY	SUNDAY
TOTAL							
GOAL							

Date: . . . .   Weight: . . . .

Breakfast

_____
_____
_____
_____

CALORIES . . . .

Lunch

_____
_____
_____
_____

CALORIES . . . .

Water

Caffeine

Dinner

_____
_____
_____
_____

CALORIES . . . .

Snacks

_____
_____
_____
_____

CALORIES . . . .

Sleep

Steps

ACTIVITY/EXERCISE	AMOUNT	NOTES

First Bite

Last Bite

My Mood is

_____
_____
_____

Ideas for Tomorrow

_____
_____
_____

Daily Calories

Date: ....   Weight: ....

Breakfast

_____
_____
_____
_____

CALORIES ....

Lunch

_____
_____
_____
_____

CALORIES ....

Dinner

_____
_____
_____
_____

CALORIES ....

Snacks

_____
_____
_____
_____

CALORIES ....

Water

Caffeine

Sleep

Steps

ACTIVITY/EXERCISE	AMOUNT	NOTES

First Bite

Last Bite

My Mood is

_____
_____
_____

Ideas for Tomorrow

_____
_____
_____

Daily Calories

Date: ....   Weight: ....

Breakfast

_____
_____
_____
_____

CALORIES ....

Dinner

_____
_____
_____
_____

CALORIES ....

Lunch

_____
_____
_____
_____

CALORIES ....

Snacks

_____
_____
_____
_____

CALORIES ....

Water

Caffeine

Sleep

Steps

ACTIVITY/EXERCISE	AMOUNT	NOTES

My Mood is

_____
_____
_____

Ideas for Tomorrow

_____
_____
_____

First Bite

Last Bite

Daily Calories

Date: ....   Weight: ....

Breakfast

_____
_____
_____
_____

CALORIES ....

Dinner

_____
_____
_____
_____

CALORIES ....

Lunch

_____
_____
_____
_____

CALORIES ....

Snacks

_____
_____
_____
_____

CALORIES ....

Water

Caffeine

Sleep

Steps

ACTIVITY/EXERCISE	AMOUNT	NOTES

My Mood is

_____
_____
_____

Ideas for Tomorrow

_____
_____
_____
_____

First Bite

Last Bite

Daily Calories

Date: ....   Weight: ....

Breakfast

_____
_____
_____
_____

CALORIES ....

Lunch

_____
_____
_____
_____

CALORIES ....

Dinner

_____
_____
_____
_____

CALORIES ....

Snacks

_____
_____
_____
_____

CALORIES ....

Water

Caffeine

Sleep

Steps

ACTIVITY/EXERCISE	AMOUNT	NOTES

My Mood is

_____
_____
_____

Ideas for Tomorrow

_____
_____
_____

First Bite

Last Bite

Daily Calories

Date: ....   **Weight:** ....

Breakfast

_____
_____
_____
_____
_____

CALORIES ....

Lunch

_____
_____
_____
_____
_____

CALORIES ....

Water

Caffeine

Dinner

_____
_____
_____
_____

CALORIES ....

Snacks

_____
_____
_____
_____

CALORIES ....

Sleep

Steps

ACTIVITY/EXERCISE	AMOUNT	NOTES

First Bite

Last Bite

My Mood is

_____
_____
_____

Ideas for Tomorrow

_____
_____
_____

Daily Calories

Date: ....   Weight: ....

Breakfast

_____
_____
_____
_____

CALORIES ....

Lunch

_____
_____
_____
_____

CALORIES ....

Dinner

_____
_____
_____
_____

CALORIES ....

Snacks

_____
_____
_____
_____

CALORIES ....

Water

Caffeine

Sleep

Steps

ACTIVITY/EXERCISE	AMOUNT	NOTES

My Mood is

_____
_____
_____

Ideas for Tomorrow

_____
_____
_____

First Bite

Last Bite

Daily Calories

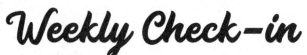

Weekly Check-in

Weekly Goals

☐ _____

☐ _____

☐ _____

Measurements

CHEST	
WAIST	
HIPS	
THIGH	
CALF	
WEIGHT	

Good Habits to Build

_____
_____
_____
_____

Bad Habits to Cut

_____
_____
_____
_____

How I'm Feeling

_____
_____
_____
_____

Reasons to keep Going

_____
_____
_____
_____

CALORIES	MONDAY	TUESDAY	WEDNESDAY	THURSDAY	FRIDAY	SATURDAY	SUNDAY
TOTAL							
GOAL							

Date: ....   Weight: ....

Breakfast

_____
_____
_____
_____

CALORIES ....

Lunch

_____
_____
_____
_____

CALORIES ....

Dinner

_____
_____
_____
_____

CALORIES ....

Snacks

_____
_____
_____
_____

CALORIES ....

Water

Caffeine

Sleep

Steps

ACTIVITY/EXERCISE	AMOUNT	NOTES

First Bite

Last Bite

Daily Calories

My Mood is

_____
_____
_____

Ideas for Tomorrow

_____
_____
_____

Date: .... Weight: ....

Breakfast

_____
_____
_____
_____
_____

CALORIES ....

Lunch

_____
_____
_____
_____
_____

CALORIES ....

Water

Caffeine

Dinner

_____
_____
_____
_____
_____

CALORIES ....

Snacks

_____
_____
_____
_____
_____

CALORIES ....

Sleep

Steps

ACTIVITY/EXERCISE	AMOUNT	NOTES

First Bite

Last Bite

My Mood is

_____
_____
_____

Ideas for Tomorrow

_____
_____
_____

Daily Calories

Date: ....   Weight: ....

Breakfast

_____
_____
_____
_____

CALORIES ....

Lunch

_____
_____
_____
_____

CALORIES ....

Dinner

_____
_____
_____
_____

CALORIES ....

Snacks

_____
_____
_____
_____

CALORIES ....

Water

Caffeine

Sleep

Steps

ACTIVITY/EXERCISE	AMOUNT	NOTES

My Mood is

_____
_____
_____

Ideas for Tomorrow

_____
_____
_____

First Bite

Last Bite

Daily Calories

Date:................. Weight:.................

Breakfast

_____
_____
_____
_____

CALORIES ....

Lunch

_____
_____
_____
_____

CALORIES ....

Dinner

_____
_____
_____
_____

CALORIES ....

Snacks

_____
_____
_____
_____

CALORIES ....

Water

Caffeine

☐ ☐ ☐
☐ ☐ ☐

Sleep

Steps

ACTIVITY/EXERCISE	AMOUNT	NOTES

First Bite

Last Bite

My Mood is

_____
_____
_____

Ideas for Tomorrow

_____
_____
_____

Daily Calories

Date:.................   Weight:.................

Breakfast

_____
_____
_____
_____

CALORIES ....

Dinner

_____
_____
_____
_____

CALORIES ....

Lunch

_____
_____
_____
_____

CALORIES ....

Snacks

_____
_____
_____
_____

CALORIES ....

Water

Caffeine

Sleep

Steps

ACTIVITY/EXERCISE	AMOUNT	NOTES

First Bite

Last Bite

My Mood is

_____
_____
_____

Ideas for Tomorrow

_____
_____
_____

Daily Calories

Date: ....   Weight: ....

Breakfast

_____

_____

_____

_____

_____

CALORIES ....

Lunch

_____

_____

_____

_____

_____

CALORIES ....

Dinner

_____

_____

_____

_____

_____

CALORIES ....

Snacks

_____

_____

_____

_____

_____

CALORIES ....

Water

Caffeine

Sleep

Steps

ACTIVITY/EXERCISE	AMOUNT	NOTES

My Mood is

_____

_____

_____

Ideas for Tomorrow

_____

_____

_____

First Bite

Last Bite

Daily Calories

Date: .... Weight: ....

Breakfast

_____
_____
_____
_____
_____

CALORIES ....

Lunch

_____
_____
_____
_____
_____

CALORIES ....

Water

Caffeine

Dinner

_____
_____
_____
_____
_____

CALORIES ....

Snacks

_____
_____
_____
_____
_____

CALORIES ....

Sleep

Steps

ACTIVITY/EXERCISE	AMOUNT	NOTES

First Bite

Last Bite

My Mood is

_____
_____
_____

Ideas for Tomorrow

_____
_____
_____
_____

Daily Calories

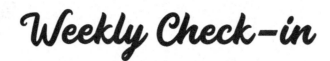

Weekly Check-in

Weekly Goals

☐ _____
_____

☐ _____
_____

☐ _____
_____

Measurements

CHEST	
WAIST	
HIPS	
THIGH	
CALF	
WEIGHT	

Good Habits to Build

_____
_____
_____
_____

Bad Habits to Cut

_____
_____
_____
_____

How I'm Feeling

_____
_____
_____
_____

Reasons to keep Going

_____
_____
_____
_____

CALORIES	MONDAY	TUESDAY	WEDNESDAY	THURSDAY	FRIDAY	SATURDAY	SUNDAY
TOTAL							
GOAL							

Date: ....

Weight: ....

Breakfast

_____
_____
_____
_____

CALORIES ....

Lunch

_____
_____
_____
_____

CALORIES ....

Water

Dinner

_____
_____
_____
_____

CALORIES ....

Snacks

_____
_____
_____
_____

CALORIES ....

Caffeine

Sleep

Steps

ACTIVITY/EXERCISE	AMOUNT	NOTES

My Mood is

_____
_____

Ideas for Tomorrow

_____
_____

First Bite

Last Bite

Daily Calories

Date: ....   **Weight:** ....

Breakfast

_____
_____
_____
_____

CALORIES ....

Lunch

_____
_____
_____
_____

CALORIES ....

Dinner

_____
_____
_____
_____

CALORIES ....

Snacks

_____
_____
_____
_____

CALORIES ....

Water

Caffeine

Sleep

Steps

ACTIVITY/EXERCISE	AMOUNT	NOTES

First Bite

Last Bite

My Mood is

_____
_____
_____

Ideas for Tomorrow

_____
_____
_____

Daily Calories

Date: ....

Weight: ....

Breakfast

_____
_____
_____
_____

CALORIES ....

Lunch

_____
_____
_____
_____

CALORIES ....

Dinner

_____
_____
_____
_____

CALORIES ....

Snacks

_____
_____
_____
_____

CALORIES ....

Water

Caffeine

Sleep

Steps

ACTIVITY/EXERCISE	AMOUNT	NOTES

My Mood is

_____
_____
_____

Ideas for Tomorrow

_____
_____
_____

First Bite

Last Bite

Daily Calories

Date: .... Weight: ....

Breakfast

_____
_____
_____
_____

CALORIES ....

Lunch

_____
_____
_____
_____

CALORIES ....

Dinner

_____
_____
_____
_____

CALORIES ....

Snacks

_____
_____
_____
_____

CALORIES ....

Water

Caffeine

Sleep

Steps

ACTIVITY/EXERCISE	AMOUNT	NOTES

My Mood is

_____
_____
_____

Ideas for Tomorrow

_____
_____
_____

First Bite

Last Bite

Daily Calories

Date: ....

Weight: ....

Breakfast

_____
_____
_____
_____

CALORIES ....

Lunch

_____
_____
_____
_____

CALORIES ....

Dinner

_____
_____
_____
_____

CALORIES ....

Snacks

_____
_____
_____
_____

CALORIES ....

Water

Caffeine

Sleep

Steps

ACTIVITY/EXERCISE	AMOUNT	NOTES

First Bite

Last Bite

My Mood is

_____
_____
_____

Ideas for Tomorrow

_____
_____
_____

Daily Calories

Date: ....   Weight: ....

Breakfast

_____
_____
_____
_____
_____

CALORIES ....

Lunch

_____
_____
_____
_____
_____

CALORIES ....

Dinner

_____
_____
_____
_____
_____

CALORIES ....

Snacks

_____
_____
_____
_____
_____

CALORIES ....

Water

Caffeine

Sleep

Steps

ACTIVITY/EXERCISE	AMOUNT	NOTES

My Mood is

_____
_____
_____

Ideas for Tomorrow

_____
_____
_____

First Bite

Last Bite

Daily Calories

Date: ....

Weight: ....

Breakfast

_____
_____
_____
_____
_____

CALORIES ....

Lunch

_____
_____
_____
_____
_____

CALORIES ....

Water

Caffeine

Dinner

_____
_____
_____
_____
_____

CALORIES ....

Snacks

_____
_____
_____
_____
_____

CALORIES ....

Sleep

Steps

ACTIVITY/EXERCISE	AMOUNT	NOTES

First Bite

My Mood is

_____
_____
_____

Ideas for Tomorrow

_____
_____
_____

Last Bite

Daily Calories

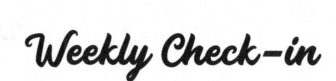

Weekly Check-in

Weekly Goals

☐ _____
_____

☐ _____
_____

☐ _____
_____

Measurements

CHEST	
WAIST	
HIPS	
THIGH	
CALF	
WEIGHT	

Good Habits to Build

_____
_____
_____

Bad Habits to Cut

_____
_____
_____

How I'm Feeling

_____
_____
_____

Reasons to keep Going

_____
_____
_____

CALORIES	MONDAY	TUESDAY	WEDNESDAY	THURSDAY	FRIDAY	SATURDAY	SUNDAY
TOTAL							
GOAL							

Date: ....

Weight: ....

Breakfast

_____
_____
_____
_____

CALORIES ....

Lunch

_____
_____
_____
_____

CALORIES ....

Dinner

_____
_____
_____
_____

CALORIES ....

Snacks

_____
_____
_____
_____

CALORIES ....

Water

Caffeine

Sleep

Steps

ACTIVITY/EXERCISE	AMOUNT	NOTES

First Bite

Last Bite

My Mood is

_____
_____
_____

Ideas for Tomorrow

_____
_____
_____

Daily Calories

Date: ....   Weight: ....

Breakfast

_____
_____
_____
_____

CALORIES ....

Lunch

_____
_____
_____
_____

CALORIES ....

Dinner

_____
_____
_____
_____

CALORIES ....

Snacks

_____
_____
_____
_____

CALORIES ....

Water

Caffeine

Sleep

Steps

ACTIVITY/EXERCISE	AMOUNT	NOTES

My Mood is

_____
_____
_____

Ideas for Tomorrow

_____
_____
_____

First Bite

Last Bite

Daily Calories

Date:.................   Weight:.................

Breakfast

_____
_____
_____
_____

CALORIES ....

Lunch

_____
_____
_____
_____

CALORIES ....

Water

Caffeine

Dinner

_____
_____
_____
_____

CALORIES ....

Snacks

_____
_____
_____
_____

CALORIES ....

Sleep

Steps

ACTIVITY/EXERCISE	AMOUNT	NOTES

First Bite

Last Bite

My Mood is

_____
_____
_____

Ideas for Tomorrow

_____
_____
_____

Daily Calories

Date: ....   Weight: ....

Breakfast

_____
_____
_____
_____

CALORIES ....

Lunch

_____
_____
_____
_____

CALORIES ....

Water

Caffeine

☐ ☐ ☐
☐ ☐ ☐

Dinner

_____
_____
_____
_____

CALORIES ....

Snacks

_____
_____
_____
_____

CALORIES ....

Sleep

Steps

ACTIVITY/EXERCISE	AMOUNT	NOTES

First Bite

My Mood is

_____
_____
_____

Ideas for Tomorrow

_____
_____
_____

Last Bite

Daily Calories

Date: ....   Weight: ....

Breakfast

_____
_____
_____
_____

CALORIES ....

Dinner

_____
_____
_____
_____

CALORIES ....

Lunch

_____
_____
_____
_____

CALORIES ....

Snacks

_____
_____
_____
_____

CALORIES ....

Water

Caffeine

Sleep

Steps

ACTIVITY/EXERCISE	AMOUNT	NOTES

First Bite

Last Bite

My Mood is

_____
_____
_____

Ideas for Tomorrow

_____
_____
_____

Daily Calories

Date: .... **Weight:** ....

Breakfast

_____
_____
_____
_____

CALORIES ....

Lunch

_____
_____
_____
_____

CALORIES ....

Water

Caffeine

Dinner

_____
_____
_____
_____

CALORIES ....

Snacks

_____
_____
_____
_____

CALORIES ....

Sleep

Steps

ACTIVITY/EXERCISE	AMOUNT	NOTES

First Bite

Last Bite

My Mood is

_____
_____
_____

Ideas for Tomorrow

_____
_____
_____

Daily Calories

Date: ....   Weight: ....

Breakfast

_____
_____
_____
_____

CALORIES ....

Lunch

_____
_____
_____
_____

CALORIES ....

Dinner

_____
_____
_____
_____

CALORIES ....

Snacks

_____
_____
_____
_____

CALORIES ....

Water

Caffeine

Sleep

Steps

ACTIVITY/EXERCISE	AMOUNT	NOTES

First Bite

Last Bite

My Mood is

_____
_____
_____

Ideas for Tomorrow

_____
_____
_____

Daily Calories

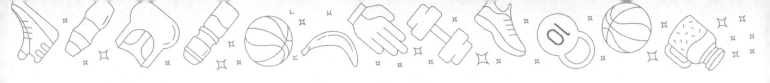

Weekly Check-in

Weekly Goals

☐ _____
_____

☐ _____
_____

☐ _____
_____

Measurements

CHEST	
WAIST	
HIPS	
THIGH	
CALF	
WEIGHT	

Good Habits to Build

_____
_____
_____
_____

Bad Habits to Cut

_____
_____
_____
_____

How I'm Feeling

_____
_____
_____
_____

Reasons to keep Going

_____
_____
_____
_____

CALORIES	MONDAY	TUESDAY	WEDNESDAY	THURSDAY	FRIDAY	SATURDAY	SUNDAY
TOTAL							
GOAL							

Date: ....

Weight: ....

Breakfast

_____
_____
_____
_____

CALORIES ....

Lunch

_____
_____
_____
_____

CALORIES ....

Water

Caffeine

Dinner

_____
_____
_____
_____

CALORIES ....

Snacks

_____
_____
_____
_____

CALORIES ....

Sleep

Steps

ACTIVITY/EXERCISE	AMOUNT	NOTES

First Bite

My Mood is

_____
_____
_____

Ideas for Tomorrow

_____
_____
_____

Last Bite

Daily Calories

Date: ....   Weight: ....

Breakfast

_____
_____
_____
_____
_____

CALORIES ....

Lunch

_____
_____
_____
_____
_____

CALORIES ....

Water

Caffeine

Dinner

_____
_____
_____
_____
_____

CALORIES ....

Snacks

_____
_____
_____
_____
_____

CALORIES ....

Sleep

Steps

ACTIVITY/EXERCISE	AMOUNT	NOTES

First Bite

My Mood is

_____
_____
_____

Ideas for Tomorrow

_____
_____
_____

Last Bite

Daily Calories

Date: .... Weight: ....

Breakfast

_____
_____
_____
_____

CALORIES ....

Lunch

_____
_____
_____
_____

CALORIES ....

Water

Caffeine

Dinner

_____
_____
_____
_____

CALORIES ....

Snacks

_____
_____
_____
_____

CALORIES ....

Sleep

Steps

ACTIVITY/EXERCISE	AMOUNT	NOTES

First Bite

My Mood is

_____
_____
_____

Ideas for Tomorrow

_____
_____
_____

Last Bite

Daily Calories

Date: ....   Weight: ....

Breakfast

_____
_____
_____
_____

CALORIES ....

Lunch

_____
_____
_____
_____

CALORIES ....

Dinner

_____
_____
_____
_____

CALORIES ....

Snacks

_____
_____
_____
_____

CALORIES ....

Water

Caffeine

☐ ☐ ☐
☐ ☐ ☐

Sleep

Steps

ACTIVITY/EXERCISE	AMOUNT	NOTES

First Bite

Last Bite

My Mood is

_____
_____
_____

Ideas for Tomorrow

_____
_____
_____

Daily Calories

Date: ....   Weight: ....

Breakfast

_____
_____
_____
_____

CALORIES ....

Lunch

_____
_____
_____
_____

CALORIES ....

Dinner

_____
_____
_____
_____

CALORIES ....

Snacks

_____
_____
_____
_____

CALORIES ....

Water

Caffeine

Sleep

Steps

ACTIVITY/EXERCISE	AMOUNT	NOTES

My Mood is

_____
_____
_____

Ideas for Tomorrow

_____
_____
_____

First Bite

Last Bite

Daily Calories

Date: ....

Weight: ....

Breakfast

_____
_____
_____
_____

CALORIES ....

Lunch

_____
_____
_____
_____

CALORIES ....

Dinner

_____
_____
_____
_____

CALORIES ....

Snacks

_____
_____
_____
_____

CALORIES ....

Water

Caffeine

Sleep

Steps

ACTIVITY/EXERCISE	AMOUNT	NOTES

My Mood is

_____
_____
_____

Ideas for Tomorrow

_____
_____
_____

First Bite

Last Bite

Daily Calories

Date: .... Weight: ....

Breakfast

_____
_____
_____
_____

CALORIES ....

Lunch

_____
_____
_____
_____

CALORIES ....

Dinner

_____
_____
_____
_____

CALORIES ....

Snacks

_____
_____
_____
_____

CALORIES ....

Water

Caffeine

Sleep

Steps

ACTIVITY/EXERCISE	AMOUNT	NOTES

First Bite

Last Bite

My Mood is

_____
_____
_____

Ideas for Tomorrow

_____
_____
_____

Daily Calories

Weekly Check-in

Weekly Goals

☐ _____
_____

☐ _____
_____

☐ _____
_____

Measurements

CHEST	
WAIST	
HIPS	
THIGH	
CALF	
WEIGHT	

Good Habits to Build

_____
_____
_____
_____

Bad Habits to Cut

_____
_____
_____
_____

How I'm Feeling

_____
_____
_____
_____

Reasons to keep Going

_____
_____
_____
_____

CALORIES	MONDAY	TUESDAY	WEDNESDAY	THURSDAY	FRIDAY	SATURDAY	SUNDAY
TOTAL							
GOAL							

Date: ....   **Weight:** ....

Breakfast

_____
_____
_____
_____
_____

CALORIES ....

Lunch

_____
_____
_____
_____
_____

CALORIES ....

Water

Caffeine

Dinner

_____
_____
_____
_____
_____

CALORIES ....

Snacks

_____
_____
_____
_____
_____

CALORIES ....

Sleep

Steps

ACTIVITY/EXERCISE	AMOUNT	NOTES

First Bite

Last Bite

My Mood is

_____
_____
_____

Ideas for Tomorrow

_____
_____
_____

Daily Calories

Date: ....   Weight: ....

Breakfast

_____
_____
_____
_____

CALORIES ....

Lunch

_____
_____
_____
_____

CALORIES ....

Dinner

_____
_____
_____
_____

CALORIES ....

Snacks

_____
_____
_____
_____

CALORIES ....

Water

Caffeine

Sleep

Steps

ACTIVITY/EXERCISE	AMOUNT	NOTES

First Bite

Last Bite

My Mood is

_____
_____
_____

Ideas for Tomorrow

_____
_____
_____

Daily Calories

Date: ....

Weight: ....

Breakfast

_____
_____
_____
_____

CALORIES ....

Lunch

_____
_____
_____
_____

CALORIES ....

Dinner

_____
_____
_____
_____

CALORIES ....

Snacks

_____
_____
_____
_____

CALORIES ....

Water

Caffeine

Sleep

Steps

ACTIVITY/EXERCISE	AMOUNT	NOTES

My Mood is

_____
_____
_____

Ideas for Tomorrow

_____
_____
_____

First Bite

Last Bite

Daily Calories

Date: ....

Weight: ....

Breakfast

_____
_____
_____
_____

CALORIES ....

Lunch

_____
_____
_____
_____

CALORIES ....

Dinner

_____
_____
_____
_____

CALORIES ....

Snacks

_____
_____
_____
_____

CALORIES ....

Water

Caffeine

Sleep

Steps

ACTIVITY/EXERCISE	AMOUNT	NOTES

My Mood is

_____
_____
_____

Ideas for Tomorrow

_____
_____
_____

First Bite

Last Bite

Daily Calories

Date: .... Weight: ....

Breakfast

_____
_____
_____
_____

CALORIES ....

Dinner

_____
_____
_____
_____

CALORIES ....

Lunch

_____
_____
_____
_____

CALORIES ....

Snacks

_____
_____
_____
_____

CALORIES ....

Water

Caffeine

Sleep

Steps

ACTIVITY/EXERCISE	AMOUNT	NOTES

First Bite

Last Bite

Daily Calories

My Mood is

_____
_____
_____

Ideas for Tomorrow

_____
_____
_____

Date: ....   **Weight:** ....

Breakfast

_____
_____
_____
_____

CALORIES ....

Dinner

_____
_____
_____
_____

CALORIES ....

Lunch

_____
_____
_____
_____

CALORIES ....

Snacks

_____
_____
_____
_____

CALORIES ....

Water

Caffeine

Sleep

Steps

ACTIVITY/EXERCISE	AMOUNT	NOTES

My Mood is

_____
_____
_____

Ideas for Tomorrow

_____
_____
_____

First Bite

Last Bite

Daily Calories

Date: ....   Weight: ....

Breakfast

_____
_____
_____
_____

CALORIES ....

Dinner

_____
_____
_____
_____

CALORIES ....

Lunch

_____
_____
_____
_____

CALORIES ....

Snacks

_____
_____
_____
_____

CALORIES ....

Water

Caffeine

Sleep

Steps

ACTIVITY/EXERCISE	AMOUNT	NOTES

First Bite

Last Bite

Daily Calories

My Mood is

_____
_____
_____

Ideas for Tomorrow

_____
_____
_____

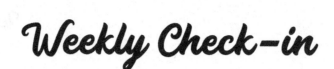

Weekly Check-in

Weekly Goals

- [ ] _____
  _____
- [ ] _____
  _____
- [ ] _____
  _____

Measurements

CHEST	
WAIST	
HIPS	
THIGH	
CALF	
WEIGHT	

Good Habits to Build

_____
_____
_____
_____

Bad Habits to Cut

_____
_____
_____
_____

How I'm Feeling

_____
_____
_____
_____

Reasons to keep Going

_____
_____
_____
_____

CALORIES	MONDAY	TUESDAY	WEDNESDAY	THURSDAY	FRIDAY	SATURDAY	SUNDAY
TOTAL							
GOAL							

Date:.................   Weight:...................

Breakfast

_____
_____
_____
_____
_____

CALORIES ....

Lunch

_____
_____
_____
_____
_____

CALORIES ....

Water

Caffeine

Dinner

_____
_____
_____
_____
_____

CALORIES ....

Snacks

_____
_____
_____
_____
_____

CALORIES ....

Sleep

Steps

ACTIVITY/EXERCISE	AMOUNT	NOTES

First Bite

Last Bite

My Mood is

_____
_____
_____

Ideas for Tomorrow

_____
_____
_____

Daily Calories

Date: ....   **Weight:** ....

Breakfast

_____
_____
_____
_____

CALORIES ....

Lunch

_____
_____
_____
_____

CALORIES ....

Water

Caffeine

Dinner

_____
_____
_____
_____

CALORIES ....

Snacks

_____
_____
_____
_____

CALORIES ....

Sleep

Steps

ACTIVITY/EXERCISE	AMOUNT	NOTES

First Bite

Last Bite

My Mood is

_____
_____
_____

Ideas for Tomorrow

_____
_____
_____

Daily Calories

Date: ....   **Weight:** ....

Breakfast

_____
_____
_____
_____

CALORIES ....

Lunch

_____
_____
_____
_____

CALORIES ....

Dinner

_____
_____
_____
_____

CALORIES ....

Snacks

_____
_____
_____
_____

CALORIES ....

Water

Caffeine

Sleep

Steps

ACTIVITY/EXERCISE	AMOUNT	NOTES

First Bite

Last Bite

Daily Calories

My Mood is

_____
_____
_____

Ideas for Tomorrow

_____
_____
_____

Date: ....

Weight: ....

Breakfast

_____
_____
_____
_____

CALORIES ....

Lunch

_____
_____
_____
_____

CALORIES ....

Dinner

_____
_____
_____
_____

CALORIES ....

Snacks

_____
_____
_____
_____

CALORIES ....

Water

Caffeine

Sleep

Steps

ACTIVITY/EXERCISE	AMOUNT	NOTES

First Bite

Last Bite

Daily Calories

My Mood is

_____
_____
_____

Ideas for Tomorrow

_____
_____
_____

Date: ....   Weight: ....

Breakfast

_____
_____
_____
_____

CALORIES ....

Lunch

_____
_____
_____
_____

CALORIES ....

Water

Caffeine

Dinner

_____
_____
_____
_____

CALORIES ....

Snacks

_____
_____
_____
_____

CALORIES ....

Sleep

Steps

ACTIVITY/EXERCISE	AMOUNT	NOTES

First Bite

My Mood is

_____
_____
_____

Ideas for Tomorrow

_____
_____
_____

Last Bite

Daily Calories

Date: .... Weight: ....

Breakfast

_____
_____
_____
_____

CALORIES ....

Lunch

_____
_____
_____
_____

CALORIES ....

Dinner

_____
_____
_____
_____

CALORIES ....

Snacks

_____
_____
_____
_____

CALORIES ....

Water

Caffeine

Sleep

Steps

ACTIVITY/EXERCISE	AMOUNT	NOTES

My Mood is

_____
_____
_____

Ideas for Tomorrow

_____
_____
_____

First Bite

Last Bite

Daily Calories

Date: ....   Weight: ....

Breakfast   ## Lunch   ## Water

_____   _____   ⬜⬜⬜⬜⬜
_____   _____   ⬜⬜⬜⬜⬜
_____   _____
_____   _____   ## Caffeine
_____   _____
CALORIES ....   CALORIES ....   ⬜ ⬜ ⬜
                                                                         ⬜ ⬜ ⬜

Dinner   ## Snacks   ## Sleep

_____   _____   [_____]
_____   _____
_____   _____   ## Steps
_____   _____
_____   _____   [_____]
CALORIES ....   CALORIES ....

ACTIVITY/EXERCISE	AMOUNT	NOTES

First Bite

[_____]

Last Bite

[_____]

My Mood is   ## Ideas for Tomorrow   ## Daily Calories

_____   _____   [_____]
_____   _____
_____   _____

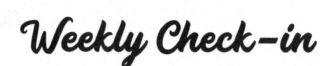

Weekly Check-in

Weekly Goals

- [ ]
- [ ]
- [ ]

Measurements

CHEST	
WAIST	
HIPS	
THIGH	
CALF	
WEIGHT	

Good Habits to Build

Bad Habits to Cut

How I'm Feeling

Reasons to keep Going

CALORIES	MONDAY	TUESDAY	WEDNESDAY	THURSDAY	FRIDAY	SATURDAY	SUNDAY
TOTAL							
GOAL							

Date: .... Weight: ....

Breakfast

_____
_____
_____
_____
_____

CALORIES ....

Lunch

_____
_____
_____
_____

CALORIES ....

Dinner

_____
_____
_____
_____

CALORIES ....

Snacks

_____
_____
_____
_____

CALORIES ....

Water

Caffeine

Sleep

Steps

ACTIVITY/EXERCISE	AMOUNT	NOTES

First Bite

Last Bite

Daily Calories

My Mood is

_____
_____
_____

Ideas for Tomorrow

_____
_____
_____
_____

Date: ....   Weight: ....

Breakfast

_____
_____
_____
_____

CALORIES ....

Lunch

_____
_____
_____
_____

CALORIES ....

Water

Dinner

_____
_____
_____
_____

CALORIES ....

Snacks

_____
_____
_____
_____

CALORIES ....

Caffeine

Sleep

Steps

ACTIVITY/EXERCISE	AMOUNT	NOTES

First Bite

Last Bite

My Mood is

_____
_____
_____

Ideas for Tomorrow

_____
_____
_____

Daily Calories

Date: ....   Weight: ....

Breakfast

_____
_____
_____
_____
_____

CALORIES ....

Lunch

_____
_____
_____
_____
_____

CALORIES ....

Water

Caffeine

Dinner

_____
_____
_____
_____
_____

CALORIES ....

Snacks

_____
_____
_____
_____
_____

CALORIES ....

Sleep

Steps

ACTIVITY/EXERCISE	AMOUNT	NOTES

First Bite

Last Bite

My Mood is

_____
_____
_____

Ideas for Tomorrow

_____
_____
_____

Daily Calories

Date: ....   Weight: ....

Breakfast

_____
_____
_____
_____

CALORIES ....

Lunch

_____
_____
_____
_____

CALORIES ....

Dinner

_____
_____
_____
_____

CALORIES ....

Snacks

_____
_____
_____
_____

CALORIES ....

Water

Caffeine

Sleep

Steps

ACTIVITY/EXERCISE	AMOUNT	NOTES	

My Mood is

_____
_____
_____

Ideas for Tomorrow

_____
_____
_____

First Bite

Last Bite

Daily Calories

Date: ....

Weight: ....

Breakfast

_____
_____
_____
_____

CALORIES ....

Lunch

_____
_____
_____
_____

CALORIES ....

Dinner

_____
_____
_____
_____

CALORIES ....

Snacks

_____
_____
_____
_____

CALORIES ....

Water

Caffeine

Sleep

Steps

ACTIVITY/EXERCISE	AMOUNT	NOTES

First Bite

Last Bite

Daily Calories

My Mood is

_____
_____
_____

Ideas for Tomorrow

_____
_____
_____

Date: ....

Weight: ....

Breakfast

_____
_____
_____
_____
_____

CALORIES ....

Lunch

_____
_____
_____
_____
_____

CALORIES ....

Dinner

_____
_____
_____
_____
_____

CALORIES ....

Snacks

_____
_____
_____
_____
_____

CALORIES ....

Water

Caffeine

Sleep

Steps

ACTIVITY/EXERCISE	AMOUNT	NOTES

My Mood is

_____
_____
_____

Ideas for Tomorrow

_____
_____
_____

First Bite

Last Bite

Daily Calories

Date:.................   Weight:.................

Breakfast

_____
_____
_____
_____

CALORIES ....

Dinner

_____
_____
_____
_____

CALORIES ....

Lunch

_____
_____
_____
_____

CALORIES ....

Snacks

_____
_____
_____
_____

CALORIES ....

Water

Caffeine

Sleep

Steps

ACTIVITY/EXERCISE	AMOUNT	NOTES

My Mood is

_____
_____
_____

Ideas for Tomorrow

_____
_____
_____

First Bite

Last Bite

Daily Calories

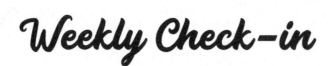

Weekly Check-in

Weekly Goals

☐ _____
_____

☐ _____
_____

☐ _____
_____

Measurements

CHEST	
WAIST	
HIPS	
THIGH	
CALF	
WEIGHT	

Good Habits to Build

_____
_____
_____
_____

Bad Habits to Cut

_____
_____
_____
_____

How I'm Feeling

_____
_____
_____
_____

Reasons to keep Going

_____
_____
_____
_____

CALORIES	MONDAY	TUESDAY	WEDNESDAY	THURSDAY	FRIDAY	SATURDAY	SUNDAY
TOTAL							
GOAL							

Date:................ Weight:.................

Breakfast

_____
_____
_____
_____

CALORIES ....

Dinner

_____
_____
_____
_____

CALORIES ....

Lunch

_____
_____
_____
_____

CALORIES ....

Snacks

_____
_____
_____
_____

CALORIES ....

Water

Caffeine

Sleep

Steps

ACTIVITY/EXERCISE	AMOUNT	NOTES

My Mood is

_____
_____
_____

Ideas for Tomorrow

_____
_____
_____

First Bite

Last Bite

Daily Calories

Date: .... Weight: ....

Breakfast

_____
_____
_____
_____

CALORIES ....

Lunch

_____
_____
_____
_____

CALORIES ....

Dinner

_____
_____
_____
_____

CALORIES ....

Snacks

_____
_____
_____
_____

CALORIES ....

Water

Caffeine

Sleep

Steps

ACTIVITY/EXERCISE	AMOUNT	NOTES

My Mood is

_____
_____

Ideas for Tomorrow

_____
_____

First Bite

Last Bite

Daily Calories

Date:................. Weight:.................

Breakfast

_____
_____
_____
_____

CALORIES ....

Lunch

_____
_____
_____
_____

CALORIES ....

Water

Caffeine

Dinner

_____
_____
_____
_____

CALORIES ....

Snacks

_____
_____
_____
_____

CALORIES ....

Sleep

Steps

ACTIVITY/EXERCISE	AMOUNT	NOTES

First Bite

My Mood is

_____
_____
_____

Ideas for Tomorrow

_____
_____
_____

Last Bite

Daily Calories

Date: ....   Weight: ....

Breakfast

_____
_____
_____
_____

CALORIES ....

Lunch

_____
_____
_____
_____

CALORIES ....

Water

Dinner

_____
_____
_____
_____

CALORIES ....

Snacks

_____
_____
_____
_____

CALORIES ....

Caffeine

Sleep

Steps

ACTIVITY/EXERCISE	AMOUNT	NOTES

First Bite

My Mood is

_____
_____
_____

Ideas for Tomorrow

_____
_____
_____

Last Bite

Daily Calories

Date:............... Weight:...............

Breakfast

_____
_____
_____
_____

CALORIES ....

Lunch

_____
_____
_____
_____

CALORIES ....

Dinner

_____
_____
_____
_____

CALORIES ....

Snacks

_____
_____
_____
_____

CALORIES ....

Water

Caffeine

Sleep

Steps

ACTIVITY/EXERCISE	AMOUNT	NOTES

My Mood is

_____
_____
_____

Ideas for Tomorrow

_____
_____
_____

First Bite

Last Bite

Daily Calories

Date: ....   **Weight:** ....

Breakfast

_____
_____
_____
_____

CALORIES ....

Lunch

_____
_____
_____
_____

CALORIES ....

Dinner

_____
_____
_____
_____

CALORIES ....

Snacks

_____
_____
_____
_____

CALORIES ....

Water

Caffeine

Sleep

Steps

ACTIVITY/EXERCISE	AMOUNT	NOTES

My Mood is

_____
_____

Ideas for Tomorrow

_____
_____

First Bite

Last Bite

Daily Calories

Date: .... Weight: ....

Breakfast

_____
_____
_____
_____
_____

CALORIES ....

Lunch

_____
_____
_____
_____
_____

CALORIES ....

Dinner

_____
_____
_____
_____
_____

CALORIES ....

Snacks

_____
_____
_____
_____
_____

CALORIES ....

Water

Caffeine

Sleep

Steps

ACTIVITY/EXERCISE	AMOUNT	NOTES

My Mood is

_____
_____
_____

Ideas for Tomorrow

_____
_____
_____

First Bite

Last Bite

Daily Calories

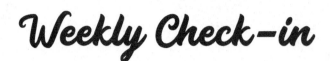

Weekly Check-in

Weekly Goals

☐ _____
_____

☐ _____
_____

☐ _____
_____

Measurements

CHEST	
WAIST	
HIPS	
THIGH	
CALF	
WEIGHT	

Good Habits to Build

_____
_____
_____
_____

Bad Habits to Cut

_____
_____
_____
_____

How I'm Feeling

_____
_____
_____
_____

Reasons to keep Going

_____
_____
_____
_____

CALORIES	MONDAY	TUESDAY	WEDNESDAY	THURSDAY	FRIDAY	SATURDAY	SUNDAY
TOTAL							
GOAL							

Date:................... Weight:...................

Breakfast

_____
_____
_____
_____

CALORIES ....

Lunch

_____
_____
_____
_____

CALORIES ....

Dinner

_____
_____
_____
_____

CALORIES ....

Snacks

_____
_____
_____
_____

CALORIES ....

Water

Caffeine

Sleep

Steps

ACTIVITY/EXERCISE	AMOUNT	NOTES

First Bite

Last Bite

Daily Calories

My Mood is

_____
_____
_____

Ideas for Tomorrow

_____
_____
_____

Date: ....   Weight: ....

Breakfast

_____
_____
_____
_____

CALORIES ....

Lunch

_____
_____
_____
_____

CALORIES ....

Dinner

_____
_____
_____
_____

CALORIES ....

Snacks

_____
_____
_____
_____

CALORIES ....

Water

Caffeine

Sleep

Steps

ACTIVITY/EXERCISE	AMOUNT	NOTES

First Bite

Last Bite

My Mood is

_____
_____
_____

Ideas for Tomorrow

_____
_____
_____

Daily Calories

Date: ....   **Weight:** ....

Breakfast

_____
_____
_____
_____
_____

CALORIES ....

Lunch

_____
_____
_____
_____
_____

CALORIES ....

Dinner

_____
_____
_____
_____
_____

CALORIES ....

Snacks

_____
_____
_____
_____
_____

CALORIES ....

Water

Caffeine

Sleep

Steps

ACTIVITY/EXERCISE	AMOUNT	NOTES

First Bite

Last Bite

My Mood is

_____
_____
_____

Ideas for Tomorrow

_____
_____
_____

Daily Calories

Date: .... Weight: ....

Breakfast

_____
_____
_____
_____

CALORIES ....

Dinner

_____
_____
_____
_____

CALORIES ....

Lunch

_____
_____
_____
_____

CALORIES ....

Snacks

_____
_____
_____
_____

CALORIES ....

Water

Caffeine

Sleep

Steps

ACTIVITY/EXERCISE	AMOUNT	NOTES

My Mood is

_____
_____
_____

Ideas for Tomorrow

_____
_____
_____

First Bite

Last Bite

Daily Calories

Date:................. Weight:.................

Breakfast

_____
_____
_____
_____
_____

CALORIES ....

Dinner

_____
_____
_____
_____

CALORIES ....

Lunch

_____
_____
_____
_____
_____

CALORIES ....

Snacks

_____
_____
_____
_____

CALORIES ....

Water

Caffeine

Sleep

Steps

ACTIVITY/EXERCISE	AMOUNT	NOTES

My Mood is

_____
_____
_____

Ideas for Tomorrow

_____
_____
_____
_____

First Bite

Last Bite

Daily Calories

Date: .... **Weight:** ....

Breakfast

_____
_____
_____
_____
_____

CALORIES ....

Lunch

_____
_____
_____
_____
_____

CALORIES ....

Dinner

_____
_____
_____
_____
_____

CALORIES ....

Snacks

_____
_____
_____
_____
_____

CALORIES ....

Water

Caffeine

Sleep

Steps

ACTIVITY/EXERCISE	AMOUNT	NOTES

My Mood is

_____
_____
_____

Ideas for Tomorrow

_____
_____
_____

First Bite

Last Bite

Daily Calories

Date:.................   Weight:.................

Breakfast

_____
_____
_____
_____
CALORIES ....

Lunch

_____
_____
_____
_____
CALORIES ....

Dinner

_____
_____
_____
_____
CALORIES ....

Snacks

_____
_____
_____
_____
CALORIES ....

Water

Caffeine

Sleep

Steps

ACTIVITY/EXERCISE	AMOUNT	NOTES

My Mood is

_____
_____
_____

Ideas for Tomorrow

_____
_____
_____
_____

First Bite

Last Bite

Daily Calories

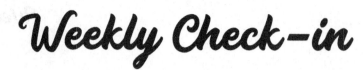

Weekly Check-in

Weekly Goals

☐ _____
_____

☐ _____
_____

☐ _____
_____

Measurements

CHEST	
WAIST	
HIPS	
THIGH	
CALF	
WEIGHT	

Good Habits to Build

_____
_____
_____
_____

Bad Habits to Cut

_____
_____
_____
_____

How I'm Feeling

_____
_____
_____

Reasons to keep Going

_____
_____
_____

CALORIES	MONDAY	TUESDAY	WEDNESDAY	THURSDAY	FRIDAY	SATURDAY	SUNDAY
TOTAL							
GOAL							

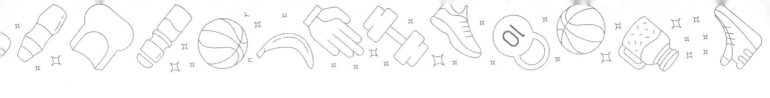

Notes

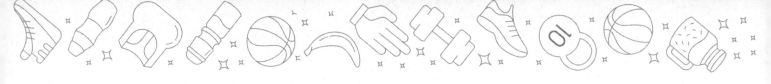

My Ending Measurements

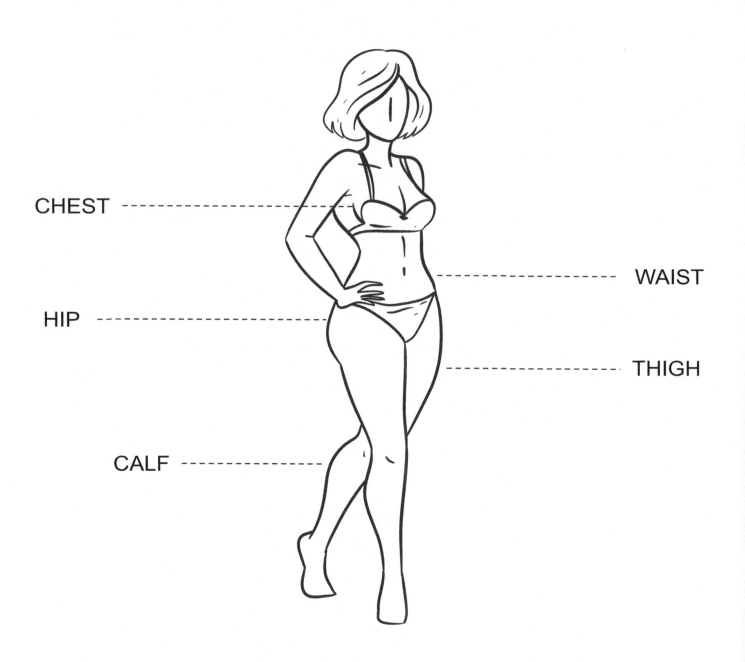

CHEST -

HIP -

CALF - - - - - - - - - - - - - -

WAIST -

THIGH - - - - - - - - - - - - - - - - - -

WEIGHT - - - - - - - - - - - - - - - - - -

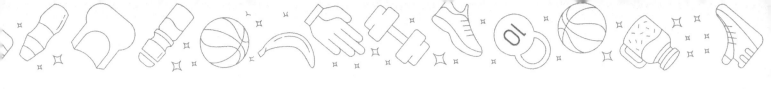

My Ending Photo

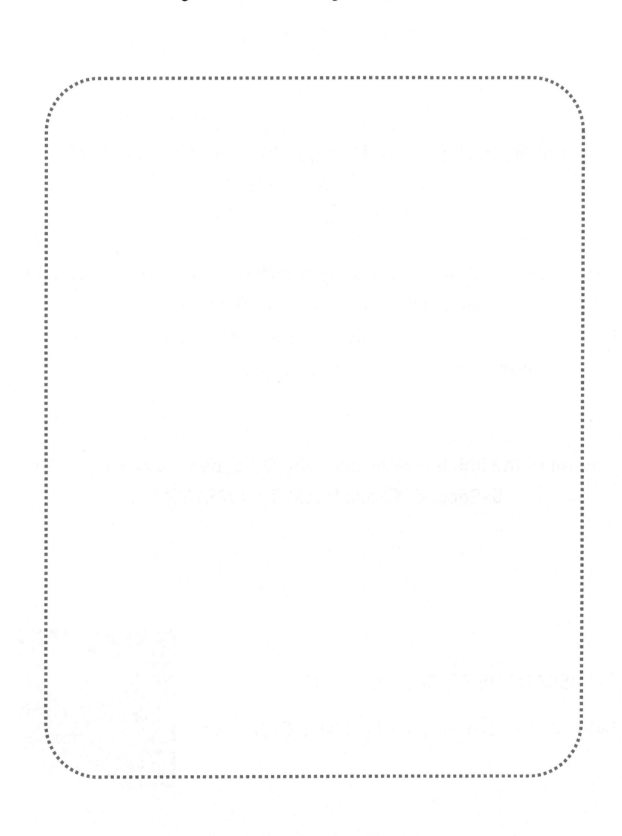

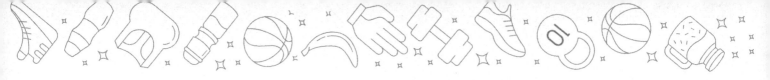

Hey there!

Are you struggling to lose weight no matter how much
you diet or exercise?
Turns out it's not your Fault

We understand that every body is different, and what works for
one person may not work for another.
That's why we want to share with you a weight loss hack that has helped
countless people shed pounds and keep them off.

Head to the link below or scan the QR code to learn about the
5-Second "Exotic Hack" That **MELTS** Fat!

SCAN THE QR CODE OR VISIT:

www.theplanetnutrition.com

Made in the USA
Las Vegas, NV
12 November 2023

80700825R00070